Dr. John K. Moore

# WEIGHT LOSS TIPS

Some useful pointers to get you started on
the path to losing weight

By

## Dr. John K. Moore

# TABLE OF CONTENTS

# Introduction

People in our society used to eat whatever their mothers made for supper, and then they went to work afterward. There was a period when the idea of being thinner never even crossed anyone's mind. The workers in that society did not have to report to a boss in the traditional sense like they do in today's society.

Individuals had to put in physical labor since there was no other option; in fact, doing so was the only way work could be done in those days. People often felt as though they could eat whatever they wanted during this time since they were burning a significantly greater number of calories than what they were taking in.

Yet, as is the case with many good things that has come to an end, and the technology of the modern world has left us in a position that might be summarized as overweight. Our life styles have

According to the proverb, "every rose has its thorn," and for our culture, the desire to have comfortable lives and to work less has begun to show around the waistline in the form of obesity.

The unfortunate thing about all of this is that the risks increase in proportion to the amount of weight you put on. If you do nothing to address your weight problem, illness of some kind, such as diabetes or a heart condition, will inevitably manifest itself in your body at some point in the future.

When it comes to putting on weight, you need to take preventative measures and keep working out until you reach a point where you no longer have any say in the matter. It's not so much about being toned and sculpted as it is about maintaining a healthy weight that won't put your life in danger. Abs are something you can work on later; right now, your primary focus should be getting rid of any excess body fat. As a culture, people are attempting to catch up and work from a position of disadvantage now that everyone is aware of what is occurring and that our nation as a whole is obese. They are making an effort to lead a better lifestyle and shed some extra pounds.

This book will serve as your guide to shedding those initial 10 pounds, which is a challenge for everyone of us. It is surprising how making a few minor adjustments to your lifestyle may result in a loss of ten pounds, and these adjustments all concentrate around eating healthily and keeping your body active.

# CHAPTER 1

# WEIGHT LOSS BEGINNING WITH WHAT YOU DRINK

Most don't aware that the first step in reducing the first 10 pounds is to change what they drink, which is a major oversight on their part. In point of fact, the vast majority of people are unaware that they may actually be dehydrated when they have feelings of hunger, and that the sensation they are having is one of thirst rather than hunger. Water is also remarkable in its own right. Water accounts for more than 66 percent of your whole body weight. This is another reason why water is such a crucial component in the process of maintaining a healthy weight. First of all, here is the TIP:

**Make sure you get lots of water**

It is recommended that you drink eight glasses of water each day; however, it may take some time for you to build up to that amount. Your body has a significant thirst and requires a lot of water. Not only does drinking water remove all of the toxins from your body, but it also helps you feel more alive, feel better and be in better health. When you drink a lot of water, you will start to feel fit almost immediately, and this will provide you with the necessary drive to lose weight.

The nicest thing about water is that it does not contain any calories, so you can drink as much of it as you like without gaining weight. When you consume a lot of water, you tend to eat less calories overall.

Always keep in mind that whenever you experience feelings of hunger, you should first drink a glass of water. After doing so, you will find that you were probably only dehydrated and not hungry at all.

You should certainly make it a goal to adhere to the regulation that recommends drinking eight glasses of water every day. Getting a jug from the pharmacy is the most reliable and accurate way to do this, as it also allows you to monitor the amount of water you consume. You can fill these up with water, then freeze them, and as the ice melts throughout the day, you'll have access to clean and cold water, making them useful aids for weight loss. You could also drink the water at room temperature if you prefer it that way and don't mind the taste difference. It is not important how much water you drink as long as you are giving your body what it needs.

**Begin each day with a clean and refreshing glass of water.**

You should have a cup of coffee or tea as soon as you get out of bed in the morning. This will assist in getting your body moving in the morning because it won't have to struggle against the effects of dehydration. In addition, if you drink a glass of water before breakfast, you won't feel as hungry and won't need to eat as much. Drinking water stimulates all of the digestive juices in your body and helps to lubricate and smooth out the digestive tract. You are more than welcome to have coffee or tea in the morning, but you should also drink a glass of water afterwards. Caffeine dehydrates you and you want to guard off dehydration.

**Have a glass of water before sitting down to eat.**

Drinking water will naturally help you feel fuller, which will result in you consuming less food overall.

**Drink some water while you are eating.**

If you drink a glass of water after each bite, you will feel fuller more quickly, which will allow you to finish your meal feeling contented rather than bloated. If you drink water as you eat, it will help your meal settle more quickly, which will in turn help you feel full more quickly.

**Avoid soda as much as possible.**

All sodas contain significant amounts of sugar for sweetening. The more you can eliminate from your diet, the better it will be for you. Additionally, diet soda is still soda. Although it may not include as much sugar as others, it does contain additional substances including components that are also detrimental to the health of your body. If you sip a Coke, you can fight back against it by drinking some water. Remember, caffeine dehydrates you as well.

Decaffeinated sodas still include trace quantities of caffeine and have the same amount of sugar as regular sodas, thus despite their name, they are not significantly more healthy. The majority of people are under the impression that fruit juice is far healthier than it actually is. The truth is that juice contains a significant amount of sugar as well. Instead of reaching for juice that has been artificially flavored and colored, satisfy your desire for a glass of juice by drinking fresh fruit juice instead. If you are able to squeeze your own fruit juice, that is even better. Be careful not to add an excessive amount of sugar, as this will raise the total number of calories. Instead of drink fruit juice, eat more fruit. Your body cannot function properly without the vitamins and fiber that fruit delivers.

**Drink less tea and coffee during the day.**

If you don't load them up with a lot of cream and sugar, they shouldn't pose much of a threat to your health. It is the sugar and cream that make the difference.

When you drink a cup of coffee or tea with cream and two cubes of sugar, you are practically eating a piece of cake. This is true whether you are drinking coffee or tea.

As long as you drink plenty of water throughout the day to counteract the effects of the caffeine that you consume, drinking black tea or coffee can actually be beneficial to your health. Caffeine is another substance that is harmful to your body.

Green tea is yet another variety of tea that can be consumed without restriction. In China, the consumption of green tea for medicinal purposes dates back more than 4,000 years. It is beneficial to the digestive system, can help relieve the discomfort of an excessively full stomach, and has been associated with a reduced risk of cancer. The best course of action would be to avoid drinking alcohol altogether if at all possible

Although moderate use of red wine may reduce the risk of coronary heart disease, the majority of alcoholic beverages are simply associated with increased body fat. Alcohol, in particular, is particularly fattening. Cocktails are fattening depending on the material that they are constructed of. Take, for example, whisky mixed with Coke. While the whiskey might not make you gain weight, the Coke most certainly will. When you're feeling a little tipsy and hungry, you won't be able to make rational decisions regarding your diet. Additionally, it's typically late at night, just before you pass out from a night of drinking, that you overeat. When you're feeling a little tipsy and hungry, you won't be able to make rational decisions regarding your diet. The overall combination is not a good one; it's just not very good.

If you absolutely have to drink alcohol, opt for a dry wine instead. You should drink dry wine rather than your wines that are higher in sugar content, because sweet wines contain more sugar. Although dry wines do contain sugar, the majority of that sugar has been fermented away into alcohol, which prevents the drinker from gaining weight.

One more thing about coffee, which isn't exactly a bad thing but is certainly more intriguing than anything else. Some individuals have stated that they were able to achieve greater weight loss when they consumed black coffee prior to engaging in physical activity. Although there is no evidence to back this up from a scientific standpoint, nutritionists believe that it may be caused by the body being forced to depend on fat as a fuel source. If you're the type of person who can drink black coffee, give it a shot.

# Chapter 2

# EATING WELL AND LOSING THE POUNDS

Yeah, so when most individuals think about shedding some pounds while maintaining their current eating habits, the word "diet" immediately comes to mind. Unfortunately, the majority of the trendy diets that are currently available lead people to put on weight over time. Why? Because they let them to starve to death, at which point the victim eventually gives in to their hunger and consumes everything in sight because they are so ravenous. In addition to this, they deny children access to the foods that they adore. This is not a healthy way to live, and it is not a healthy way to lose weight. You are the only one who gives oneself tension, and stress is the underlying cause of your weight increase!

Thus, if you want to eat healthily, there are a few guidelines that you should follow each and every day. These guidelines will not prevent you from eating the meals that you enjoy, but they will teach you to view such foods as luxuries so that you may appreciate them even more.

Consume plenty of fresh fruits and vegetables, as these foods contain a high proportion of water. Tomatoes, watermelons, cantaloupe, kiwis, and grapes are some examples of these types of foods. You get the picture. You should eat a lot of those luscious fruits and vegetables because they are fresh and full of taste. These foods contain an average of 90–95% water, which means that you may consume a large quantity of them without gaining any additional weight even if they are quite filling.

**Consume fresh fruit rather than processed varieties of fruit.**

Something that is transformed into additional sugar during processing. Moreover, canned and processed fruits do not have the same amount of fiber content as fresh fruits.

Increase your consumption of fiber to the greatest extent you are able to. In most cases, this entails increasing the amount of fruit and vegetables consumed.

When it comes to getting rid of excess fat, is that vegetables are your best allies. Because there are so many options available to you right now, you might be interested in sampling ones that you haven't tried in the past. The leafy green varieties are the best, and you should try to incorporate as many of them as possible into your salads. As long as you don't drown them with dressing and pile on too much cheese, salads are an excellent source of a wide variety of vitamins and minerals. The leafy greens contain a significant amount of natural water as well.

**Make informed decisions about the food that you consume.**

Do not eat for the sake of eating. People only eat when they are aware that their bodies truly require it, but animals eat because it is in their nature to do so. Eat less on the spur of the moment.

Be mindful of everything you put into your body, from the food itself to the condiments you put on it. Because most condiments and garnishes include a lot of fat, they have the potential to ruin an otherwise nutritious meal.

This does not mean that you cannot enjoy sweets; nonetheless, you should avoid eating them in place of a meal. Always keep in mind that eating these sweets will eventually contribute to an area in which you do not want them to contribute. Yet, you should not deprive yourself, since this will cause you to consume twice as many as what is healthy for you.

**Establish meal times and keep to them per recommendation.**

Make it a goal to eat all of your meals at the times that you have scheduled for them. Developing a regular eating routine will assist you in maintaining better control over the foods and times that you consume them. Also, rather than eating just one or two extremely large meals per day, it is recommended that you have a total of five smaller meals each day. If you just eat once a day, your body will think it is starving and will store fat instead of using it as fuel because it only gets food once a day. In addition, you shouldn't wait until you're ravenous before eating something. This will just cause you to overeat until you are completely full.

Eat just when you feel like it, which is tip number 21. Be sure to start by having a glass of water so that you can assess whether or not you are actually thirsty or hungry before continuing. When confronted with food, a lot of people can't help but stuff their faces. It does not imply that they are hungry; rather, they simply desire to consume it. If you're not hungry, you shouldn't consume anything that's presented to you.

Make it a goal to avoid snacking in the time between meals, but if you absolutely must have something to eat, choose for a nutritious option. If you travel a lot, you should look for healthy snacks rather than junk food to eat on the road.

**Veggies make terrific snacks.**

They have the ability to help you over the feelings of hunger if you are experiencing them. Carrots are wonderful both for their ability to sate hunger and for the abundance of nutrients that they contain.

When it comes to those foods that you simply cannot live without, keeping track of the calories you consume is a smart idea. If it is a pre-packaged food item, then the nutritional information, including the number of calories, will be printed on the packaging. Be sure to keep an eye on the calorie content as well as the serving size when making your selections.

Get in some extra exercise before the weekend so you can burn off those extra calories.

If you feel like you've overindulged this week, be sure to get to the gym or walk for a bit longer so that you can burn off the additional calories you've consumed.

Avoid eating anything that has been fried at all costs. If it has breading, baking is the preferred preparation method. Fried dishes are doused in fat and oil during the cooking process. There is still oil absorbed into the food item itself after the surplus oil has been drained away, even though there is less oil in the food item overall.

**Don't skip meals.**

You ought to consume at the very least three meals per day, but the optimal number is five relatively little meals. Because of this, you won't find yourself starving throughout the day and end up eating more than you need to as a result.

**Similar to fruits, fresh veggies are superior than their canned counterparts.**

If you are able to consume your vegetables in their raw form, that is ideal. As you heat foods, many of the beneficial nutrients are destroyed. If you absolutely must cook them, the best way to do it is to boil them for a short period of time until they retain some of their crispness. Additionally, you shouldn't let the butter melt into them. It is preferable to purchase vegetables that are organic and untreated with pesticides whenever possible.

**Eat only one egg per day at the most**

It would be ideal if you could limit your consumption of eggs to no more than three per week.

Chocolates are considered luxury commodities and should be treated as such. Purchase items of higher quality and limit your consumption of them to infrequent occasions. If you take the time to appreciate each bite, you'll find that the act of eating brings you much more pleasure, and the food will be even more satisfying as a result.

Be sure that your daily diet includes items from each of the different food categories. This is an excellent method for ensuring that your body receives all of the nutrients it need, and it also helps to ward off any dietary shortages that may exist. Also, try to vary the foods you consume on a regular basis. Try new things so that you won't get used to the same old diet and become bored.

Aim to consume breakfast within the first hour of waking up in the morning. This is the most effective method for providing your body with the kickstart it requires. Avoid waiting until you are extremely hungry before eating.

Although though breakfast is a very important meal, there is no need to overindulge. The concept behind this is that you have gone without eating all night long, and now you are breaking your fast.

Your diet should incorporate all aspects of the food groups, including carbohydrates, in order to be considered balanced. Your diet should actually consist of roughly 50–55% carbohydrates.

Carbohydrates are an excellent source of fuel. Diets that restrict carbohydrate consumption are not only ineffective but also harmful since they make people crave carbohydrates even more. Your diet should not lead you to lack any essential nutrients in any way.

You should limit the amount of protein in your diet to between 25 and 30 percent. There is an excessive amount of focus placed on meat as the primary component of your meal. In point of fact, one would be better off considering it more of an accompaniment rather than the primary course.

Between 15 and 20 percent of your daily calorie intake ought to come from fats. This amount of fat is actually all that is required by your body. The likes of milk, sugar, and other similar substances are going to make up a significant portion of this in your diet.

Consume more white meat and less red meat, as this is the 36th helpful hint. Chicken, fish, and various other fowl are all examples of white flesh. Beef and pork are both examples of red meat.

If you can, transition to a vegetarian diet entirely. Even if you are unable to entirely give up meat, you will still be leading a better life by adopting this lifestyle. The more fruits and vegetables you can consume, the better it will be for you. The less meat you eat, the less fat you need to consume in order to maintain your current weight. But, since protein is essential, you need to make sure that the alternative you choose enables you to keep up a healthy level of protein consumption.

Bread should be consumed in moderation, and while white bread is fine, high-fiber multigrain breads are far superior.

These breads are an additional option to add more fiber to your diet, and in addition, they contain a sufficient amount of protein.

Pork does not in any way facilitate weight loss, so steer clear of it if you're trying to trim down. When you are aiming to reduce the amount of weight you are carrying, eating less pork will help you do better. Pork products, which include fatty meats like bacon, ham, and sausage, have a high percentage of total fat.

**Decrease the amount of sugar you consume.**

If you really have to put something sweet in your coffee and tea, experiment with several flavors of artificial sweetener until you discover one that suits your palate. However, these things are not particularly nutritious either and should be consumed in moderation just like the others.

Try eating smaller meals more frequently throughout the day. These are the bite-sized meals that we talked about earlier on. Some people are more successful at losing weight when they never feel hungry, and grazing on nutritious food items can help you accomplish this goal. In addition to this, it maintains your metabolism active, which in turn burns fat in a natural way.

Do not be concerned about cheating, but do not cheat in order to obtain food.

Consume sweets and your go-to cheat meal solely for the flavor they provide. If you still have room for dessert after dinner, offer to split one with the rest of the family. You won't put on weight while enjoying the delicious flavor.

**Watch how much fat you eat**

There are 9 calories in every gram of fat. You will be able to calculate the quantity of fat in those goods if you know the total number of calories they contain.

Go easy on the salt and attempt to reduce the amount you use by half. One of the most important contributors to the obesity epidemic is salt.

Dr. John K. Moore

# Chapter 3

# LOSE WEIGHT BY CHANGING HOW YOU COOK

Modifying how you cook your meals is one of the easiest ways to shed those first ten pounds, and the following are some suggestions that will help you do just that. The manner in which food is prepared has an equal amount of influence on whether or not it is healthful.

If you want to avoid the health risks associated with frying in oil or fat, try baking the food instead. Baking does not require as much grease and oil as frying does, and the food does not absorb any of those ingredients as it cooks thanks to baking's dry heat.

If you want to avoid using oil, spray your frying pan with non-stick cooking spray. Moreover, cooking using pans that do not stick requires significantly less oil, if any at all.

Instead of cooking vegetables, try boiling them beforehand. You might also steam them, which is said to be the healthiest preparation method for veggies such as cauliflower, cabbage, and broccoli.

Be wary of food items labeled as having no fat or low fat content. There is a large selection of these food items available to buy, but they are not really nutritious in any way. In order to get the desired level of sweetness in many of these food products, various types of chemicals or carbohydrates are used.

On the other hand, these chemicals and carbohydrates are converted into sugar by the body, which means that they continue to be metabolized into fat even after being consumed.

**Do not make the mistake of going on a crash diet.**

They are not beneficial for you and, in the long run, will cause more harm than good to your health. The short-term effects often include a loss of a few pounds; but, once you stop using them, all of your weight will return, and it will be higher than it was before. Crash diets are not sustainable in the long run, so you will inevitably reach a point where you have no choice but to abandon them.

**Use a high-quality Extra Virgin Olive Oil if you are cooking with oil.**

It is more expensive than vegetable oil; nevertheless, the health benefits it provides are significantly superior, making the higher cost worthwhile. Olive oil has been linked to a lower incidence of coronary heart disease, and it also helps to strengthen the suppleness of arterial walls, both of which can help lower blood pressure.

# Chapter 4

# EXERCISING TO SEE RESULTS IN WEIGHT LOSS

There are two things that you must do in order to lose weight, and one of those things is eating properly and filling your body with good, clean water. We have already covered the first of these two things rather extensively, so let's move on to the second. Get your body moving, as it is the second thing you have to do to succeed.

It is not necessary to sign up for a membership at a gym in order to work out. In point of fact, there are a number of things that you can do on a daily basis that will assist in getting your career off the ground.

When you first start working out, whether you do it at home or in a gym, try not to get disheartened if you don't notice results right away. It takes more than a week for your body to get into shape, which is necessary before you can start making progress. Although it just takes a short amount of time to see results from their workouts, many people make the mistake of believing that their workouts are ineffective.

When you initially start working out, it's important not to put too much pressure on your body or you run the risk of injuring yourself. Your skeletal system, including your joints and ligaments, is not ready for the amount of strain you are putting on it. It is a mistake to believe that you will shed pounds simply by working out more intensely for a shorter period of time; the human body simply does not function in this manner. When it comes to physical activity, doing things slowly and steadily is the best strategy.

Check your weight before you start exercising, but don't take that as a measurement of how much weight you're going to lose from doing so. Your weight is prone to going up and down throughout the day. If you check your weight every day, you run the risk of becoming disheartened with your progress.

The fit of your clothes is the best indicator of whether or not you are successfully reducing weight. If you start to feel as though you are floating in your clothes, then you can be sure that the food you are consuming and the exercise you are doing are helping you. One further way to tell whether you're getting thinner is if you notice that you're able to move the spot where you normally buckle your belt; obviously, a tighter fit is preferable.

Reward yourself after conducting periodic checks of your weight and the way in which your clothes fit. You should treat yourself to a new pair of trousers and some new running shoes. This will assist you in maintaining your motivation as you work toward achieving your weight loss goals.

Give your body a break from your workout routine once in a while so that it may relax and rebuild itself. One day of rest each week is necessary for your body.

Exercising for thirty minutes on three days of the week can help you maintain your current weight; however, in order to start losing weight, you need to exercise for thirty minutes on at least four days of the week; five days of the week is optimal.

 Compile information on simple exercises and other activities that may be done from the comfort of your own home. There is a vast amount of information that is currently available on exercise, and you can select what will be most helpful to you in achieving your objectives about weight loss. Look up information about health and exercise on the Internet or pick up some books at your neighborhood bookstore or library to obtain additional information and guidance on how to burn the ideal quantity of calories that you have set for yourself to burn each week.

Look for a workout partner. This should be someone who is as qualified as they are committed to working out and reducing weight in the same way that you are. One of the advantages of finding a partner who is willing to commit to you is that you will always have someone to share your feelings with.

The awareness that there is someone else looking forward to seeing you makes it your ability to get out of bed and go exercise with them will be facilitated. You wouldn't want to be the person to ditch your workout partner, would you?

Listen to your body and stop what you're doing when it tells you it's had enough. After a significant amount of time spent exercising, your body will begin sending you signals to let you know how it feels about the workout. This is especially crucial when you are first beginning an exercise routine because it will help you avoid injury.

If you decide to extend the duration of your workouts, make sure to do so in a measured and controlled manner. The same is true with regard to the level of difficulty of your workouts.

Choose an exercise routine that is appropriate for your lifestyle. Everyone lives their life a little differently and goes about their day doing something a little bit different. There is no fixed time during which you should or should not engage in physical activity. If you find that working out late at night before going to bed helps you unwind and is enjoyable to you, then you should continue to do so. If you find that getting some exercise in the morning helps you get your day started on the right foot, then it's a terrific habit to have. Some people find that doing out during their lunch break is an effective way to relieve the stress caused by their jobs, while others do it because it is the only time they have available.

**Do not just stand about; instead, move around.**

If you are able to move around, then you should do so. Individuals who walk at a steady pace are actually doing themselves a lot of favors by staying active and keeping their bodies in motion. Also, playing helps you think more clearly.

Do not sit if you are able to stand instead. If you are able to stand for long periods of time without becoming fatigued, you will expend more calories doing so than sitting would.

The couch and the television are both bad for your efforts to lose weight. If you have a tendency to become a couch potato, resist the urge to sit on the sofa. In point of fact, if you really must, add a not so

Provide a chair that provides sufficient comfort in front of the television in the hopes that you will watch it less frequently. If you're addicted to the computer in the same way, the same advice applies to you. There are some people who have a chair in front of their computer that is more comfortable than the one they have in front of their television. (Of course, this only applies if you don't work from home and have to sit in front of your computer for long stretches at a time, in which case having a comfortable chair is quite crucial.)

If you have a work that requires you to sit the entire time, make sure to get up and stretch at least once every half an hour. The vast majority of occupations available in this day and age involve working in front of a computer and need you to sit down. If you have this kind of job, you should make it a point to switch locations at regular intervals.

Get up and move around while you're talking on the phone. If it is a lengthy discussion, you will have a fantastic opportunity to work on your fitness.

The 69th helpful hint is to take the stairs rather than the elevator or escalator. They are wonderful conveniences, yet they cause us to become quite sluggish and unproductive. Using the stairs instead of waiting for the elevator to become available is another time-saving option.

**Stop smoking.**

Although smoking doesn't directly affect your weight, it might cause irregular eating patterns and make you more dependent on coffee.

Ten minutes of cardiovascular activity every day is optimal for most people; you can fulfill this need through activities other than jogging.

 If you are unable to run due to a physical condition, you can maintain your fitness by going for a brisk stroll for 15 minutes.

If you have enough time, you can walk almost anyplace. If your place of employment or the supermarket is not too far away, you might want to think about walking or riding your bike there. Even if it will take you a little longer, at least you will be working out during that time.

If you want to fool yourself, hide the remote control. When it comes to slimming down, remote controllers are just as bad as fast food. You might not even be able to switch on the television if you didn't have the remote, which implies you might look for more physically demanding activities to do instead.

Instead than sitting in front of the television and watching it, you should get up and manually change the channel if you don't have a remote, or go for a walk.

**Doing your own fetching**

Walk and get it yourself if you need something from the kitchen, want to change the channel on the television, fetch the mail or the newspaper from the driveway, etc. It will do you a world of good to incorporate some walking into your daily routine.

**Take the stairs, walk along the escalator, or use it to help you ascend the steps.**

At the time that the show is taking a commercial break, get up and move around or perform some basic exercises such as crunches or bending over and touching your toes. Try everything you can to increase the amount of movement your body makes and to keep your blood pumping throughout the day.

**Put on some music and dance.**

To reiterate, the more you move about, the better you'll feel overall, and the more weight you'll lose.

If you are on public transit, get off one block before your stop, and then walk the remaining distance to your destination. This provides a convenient opportunity to get in a walk before and after work, as well as on the route to or from another location.

**Do pelvic gyrations in order to prepare for your midsection exam.**

It goes without saying that you wouldn't perform these in front of anyone, but they are a beneficial stage in the process of getting your body ready for more intense abdominal crunches. It is also beneficial for the muscles in your back, and it prevents you from being tight rather of keeping you flexible.

When you walk, pull your tummy in toward your spine. Walk normally, but make an effort to pull your stomach in against your spine at all times. You should start to feel those muscles contracting in the very near future.

To tone your abdominal muscles, try doing some breathing exercises. It is incredible to see how

It's a little-known fact, but breathing correctly and engaging your whole diaphragm can actually help you tone your abdominal muscles. Indeed, the majority of individuals have poor breathing habits, and the brain benefits from adequate oxygen intake.

**Try with yoga.**

Weight loss and stress relief are two of the many benefits that can be attained via regular yoga practice. You will learn how to regulate your muscles and gain more control over each particular group of your muscles when you practice yoga.

**Lift weights.**

People tend to underestimate the amount of fat that can be burned when they strength exercise. When people work on increasing their muscular mass, they start to lose fat in order to fuel their growing muscles. Be aware that if you increase your muscle mass, the scale may no longer be an accurate tool for determining whether or not you have lost weight. This is because muscle weighs more than fat does.

**Massage your companion.**

You can push yourself a little bit, and if they have been working out with you, you will also be able to congratulate them on the weight loss they have achieved, which will allow you to do both at the same time.

Climb the stairs two at a time rather than one at a time. Because of this, you will need to push yourself more, which will cause your heart rate to increase.

**Take your dog on a walk.**

If you don't get enough exercise, it's likely that neither does your pet. This is especially true if you have a larger pet. Or, you may allow your dog lead the way on your walk. Let him take charge of the situation for once in his life and allow him decide where he wants to go and how quickly he wants to get there. You and your partner might benefit physically by participating in this activity.

**Take a dancing lesson.**

This may take the form of ballroom dancing, in which popular dances such as the tango, salsa, and fox trot are taught. These dances have a quick tempo, and they are designed to get you moving. Even at a medium tempo, ballroom dancing is a vigorous activity that will

Definitely work on your leg muscle tone. Or, you may enroll in a dancing fitness class. How many dancers do you know who are considerably heavier than they should be?

The wall should be leant against such that your face is near to it, and then you should use your hands to push your body away from the wall. Do this stretching exercise three or four times.

**Swim whenever the opportunity presents itself.**

Those who suffer from osteoporosis or other joint conditions will find that swimming offers a fantastic opportunity to get their cardiac workout in while having little to no negative impact on their joints.

**Playing tennis or basketball.**

Getting into the spirit of shape can be accomplished quite well by playing games. Working out with another person in a setting that encourages healthy competition is not only more effective but also more pleasant.

You should always begin your workout with a warm-up that lasts approximately 5-10 minutes, and you should always complete your workout with a cool-down that lasts about 5-10 minutes. Before the rest of the workout, your body has to attain a particular heart rate level before it will respond well to the exercises.

Do not bring your wireless phone or cell phone with you anywhere. If it rings, you should go get it by foot. There are a lot of helpful things in life, and we almost always have everything we require right at our fingertips, but obviously this is not good for the size of our waistlines.

If you're going to be standing around for a while, try stretching your legs a little bit by standing on your toes for a moment and then lowering yourself slowly to your heels. Moreover, you can flex your buttocks muscles as well, albeit perhaps only when no one else is around to see it.

**Take some time to examine your appearance in the mirror while you are naked before going to bed**

Note the aspects of your performance that require improvement as well as those that highlight your strengths. Keeping yourself motivated during your workout might be helped along by conducting a self-inventory endeavors. Additionally, don't forget to compliment yourself on any improved muscle tone or other improvements you may have made in your life. This is really important.

**Do not slump in your chair.**

At all times, you should make an effort to sit up straight and tall. When you slouch, not only is it unhealthy for your back, but it also makes you seem fat. Always make it a priority to maintain proper sitting and standing posture.

The vast majority of people would prefer to focus on their stomachs and get rid of that area entirely as their primary goal. We are unable to perform spot reductions, unfortunately. Yet, one thing you can do to assist tighten the muscles in your stomach is to engage in a breathing exercise.

Take a deep breath in and try to make it as powerful as you can while simultaneously pulling in your stomach as much as you can. Keep your grip on it for a couple of seconds, and then slowly let it go. Don't let it out so quickly that your stomach comes tumbling out. This is a really bad sign. Make an effort to breathe in this manner anytime you remember to do so, ideally between 50 and 60 times per day. You should expect to drop at least half an inch after following this plan for approximately twenty days.

Employ a chart to help you with your efforts to lose weight, like the one that is provided for you below. This chart provides an estimate of how many calories can be burned by performing a variety of common activities for a period of twenty minutes.

# Chapter 5

# GETTING STARTED

Now that you know how to get started, here is some further information on how to lose weight and keep it off, and it all starts with what you put in your mouth.

Because we are fatter now than we have ever been before, getting rid of excess fat and weight is a very vital part of our lives today. Anyone who is eavesdropping on a conversation or watching television will immediately become interested when they hear the phrase "weight loss programs."

In point of fact, that is currently one of the most frequently searched-for keywords on the internet.

Our relationship with food is the primary contributor to our nation's epidemic of obesity and overeating. In our culture, there is a predisposition to place an emphasis on quantity. Instead of wanting the best food that we can get our hands on, all we want is as much as we can obtain. In every situation, quantity is prioritized over quality, despite the fact that this should be exactly the reverse of the case.

When you've made the decision to shed some pounds, the next step can be figuring out where to start.

You ought to get the ball rolling right away. It is possible to get moving and reduce weight, but only if you have a firm determination to do it. You only need to practice your refusal to comply with requests.

Everybody is different. You won't find another individual who has the same metabolism as you have or who burns fat in the same manner as you do. No one else will have either of those things. You may

You and the person next to you might weigh the same amount, but if you both started an exercise and diet regimen, you might not have the same outcomes two weeks or even a month later, even if you did everything the exact same way each time.

In light of this, it is essential to be aware that not everyone makes the same kind of use of the food they consume. Anything that makes one individual gain a pound could not have the same effect on another person. The same is true for getting rid of excess weight. If you are a married woman and you and your husband are working out together, and let's say that he stops drinking soda and loses five pounds as a result of cutting back on his consumption of soda, but you don't lose any weight as a result of giving up soda, what does that mean?

Simply said, people in today's society are expected to put in significantly more effort than their ancestors did at the same level of productivity. When we look back sixty years, both men and women were physically fit because they had to work hard. You were expected to perform manual labor or else you wouldn't be able to eat. If you wanted eggs, you had to go collect them from the hen house. If you wanted fresh milk, you had to go milk the cows.

If you wanted to cultivate your own veggies, you had to plough the fields. If you wanted beef, you had to be at least a little bit knowledgeable about how to raise a calf to maturity and then have it killed. That was how life was back then, but thanks to advances in technology, most of the manual labor has been eliminated. So, we need to pay attention to what we put in our bodies and ensure that we get plenty of physical activity.

It is very vital to have a clear understanding that the success of your efforts to lose weight is highly dependent on the amount of effort that you are willing to put in. If you want to succeed in this one area of your life, you will have to put in a lot of hard work if you want to see results.

People typically do not need to be concerned about their weight until they reach their twenties; but, due to the fast food lifestyle that many of us live today, this is not necessarily the case anymore. Because they consume an excessive amount of fast food and processed meals, many of our youngsters are overweight. Read the labels on the foods you and your family buy at the grocery store to ensure that you are getting what you expect from them. If you can't say the word, you can't say it.

Do not consume it. Processed foods are to blame for our insatiable appetites, which, in turn, contribute to our weight gain. If you ever want to be successful at losing weight and keeping it off, it is especially vital to understand why this happens and how to prevent it.

But, paying attention to your nutrition won't be enough to cause weight loss on its own. In addition to maintaining an appropriate diet, one also needs to get the recommended quantity of physical activity. The solution is to develop an exercise routine that will provide your body with the necessary amount of physical activity.

If you do not move, it is the same as if you were in hibernation, and your body will just pack on the pounds, especially in the area around your midsection.

When you think of life in the past, when your sweat was created by hard labor and the sun, it just makes you feel wonderful all over. This is because your sweat was a sign that you were living a healthy lifestyle. You feel physically stronger all over as a result of the sun pounding down on your shoulders and the strain that the strain puts on your muscles.

There is just nothing that can compare to working out in the fresh air.

Yet, the majority of people now live in urban areas. It has been a long time since most people had the opportunity to work on a farm; yet, there are a select few who are able to continue to experience the exhilarating sensation of being productive while simultaneously avoiding the accumulation of extra weight thanks to their chosen occupation. If you really give it some thought, how many farm hands, cowboys, and ranchers do you think are overweight? There aren't very many of them. Consider the way they live their lives.

They get up, have some coffee and breakfast, go to work, come back for lunch, go back to work, come back for dinner, and then they go to bed at an appropriate hour so that they can get up for work the next day get up in the morning and repeat the process from the beginning. In the meantime, they soak up the sun, breathe in the crisp air, and drink plenty of clean water throughout the day. It is, in every sense of the word, a healthy way of life. Unfortunately, most of us work indoors, sitting down, and we still have to eat three meals a day, but we have to do it so quickly that we don't even get the chance to taste what we're eating.

Unless you live in a metropolis where you walk everywhere you go, it is a sad reality that people who live in the city don't get nearly as much physical activity as those who live in the suburbs. This indicates that you need to set your mind to it and put in the effort to achieve your goals. You have to make time in your schedule for physical activity every day; else, you will end up being overweight and sick. That has to be accepted as the truth. The most effective method for preventing and treating obesity, as well as stress, hypertension, and cardiovascular disease, is regular physical activity. The ability to complete your workout outside is ideal. Your body requires an abundance of clean air in whatever form it can find it.

Maintaining a steady pace throughout an exercise routine is the single most important factor in its success. If you have a goal in mind, and you work toward that goal on a consistent basis, you will eventually be able to achieve that goal.

People typically have little difficulty getting started. They go shopping, purchase some training clothes and running shoes, and may even sign up for a membership at a local gym. After that, they go to the gym and work out very consistently for the next week or two.

Yet as time goes on, they discover that it becomes increasingly difficult to stick to their regimen. As the demands of their lives increase, they find that they have less time to devote to going to the gym. In other words, people simply quit attending to the gym, which means that their gym subscription is wasted.

Although though nighttime exercise is something that a lot of people do, maintaining a consistent regimen can be challenging for some people. If you are not totally worn out when you get home from work, then now would be a good time to leave. If you are unable to, though, you will need to figure out how to get there first thing in the morning. It will assist you in waking up, and you will be able to keep your consistency intact as a result of doing so.

There is a common belief that physical activity will leave you feeling exhausted, however this might not always be the case. It is possible that the first few times it does this to you, but as you continue to get fit, you will notice that you have more energy. If you combine your workouts with getting enough rest, you shouldn't have any trouble getting out of bed in the morning and getting things done. In addition to this, you will maintain your energy levels throughout the day, which will make it much simpler for you to go through your workday.

Even if you don't have a subscription to a gym, there is a good possibility that there is a sidewalk outside your house, and some individuals may even have access to a pool. Even if you don't have a gym membership, you can still get some exercise. Wake up a half an hour early, lace on your shoes, and begin your chosen kind of cardio immediately—whether it's walking, running, jogging, or something else. If you have a furry companion, they will most likely enjoy spending time with you just as much as you will.